Tibetan Healing Science

Bod Kyi Sowa Rigpa

Tibetan Healing Science

Bod Kyi Sowa Rigpa

Dr Pema Dorjee

with Eleanor Lincoln Morse

Fox Print Books

Published by: Fox Print Books
45 Pleasant Ave
Peaks Island, ME 04108
foxprintbooks@gmail.com
207.766.3335

Contents

8

Dedicated to our loving mother,
the late Mrs. Norbu Dolma

10

Keeping your body healthy is an expression of gratitude to the whole cosmos— the trees, the clouds, everything.

Thich Nhat Hanh — Vietnamese Buddhist monk, poet and peace activist

1

INTRODUCTION

This primer on Tibetan healing science was laid out in a series of meetings in 2008. While living in northern India during 2006, Eleanor Morse first met Dr. Pema Dorjee, a renowned practitioner of Tibetan Medicine and Director of the Research Department at Men-Tsee-Khang, the Tibetan Medical and Astrological Institute in Dharamsala, India. Together, they discussed the possibility of a joint writing project which would help make information about the benefits of Tibetan medicine more accessible to Westerners. Dr. Dorjee, who has been practicing Tibetan medicine for over thirty years, seeing hundreds of patients a year, is in a unique position to bring Tibetan Healing Science to the West. As an expert practitioner, he has lectured at universities on several continents, helping to create a bridge that furthers understanding between worlds.

Over a three-week period in February of 2008, Eleanor met with Dr. Dorjee after he'd finished seeing patients for the day. As the sun set over the Dhauladhar Mountains just beyond the porch, they began each session with a cup of tea poured by Tenzin Choeying, Pema Dorjee's youngest daughter, who had just finished her own medical training at the Tibetan Medical College in Dharamsala. A special thanks to her. She has been invaluable during this project, helping to translate Dr. Dorjee's ideas into English and making suggestions about additions to the manuscript.

What follows is intended as a contribution toward helping East and West to join hands in providing as wide a spectrum of health care as possible to patients in need of healing.

2

THE FOUNDATION OF TIBETAN MEDICINE

HISTORY

Over the centuries, the geography of Tibet has contributed to the development of a culture and a form of Buddhism unique to the region. With an average elevation of over 16,000 feet, Tibet is the highest region on Earth, a country of soaring peaks and high lakes and plateaus; for thousands of years, it was close to impenetrable.

In the 4th century or earlier, Tibetan medical practitioners were influenced by early forms of Ayurvedic medicine practiced in India. Beginning in the 7th and 8th centuries, influences reached Tibet from Persia, Greece and China. Around the 11th century, a mosaic of medical thinking was codified into a system of Tibetan medicine and imbued with a Buddhist framework that expressed the relationship between body and mind and the individual's connection to the natural world.

Tibetan medicine, or the Healing Science of Tibet (*Bod kyi sowa rigpa*), emphasizes the body's natural balance and instinct for health. Over time, Tibetan medical practitioners developed sophisticated methods for the diagnosis and treatment of illness that did not require numbers, technology, or the objectification and reduction of observations to capturable data. Practitioners used what was available to them: listening, observation, and intuition honed by experience and intensive training.

Beginning with a foundation of Buddhist philosophy which encouraged a clear, wise, unobstructed mind and a compassionate heart, physicians learned to read the complexities of a patient's physical, mental and psychological being, to listen intently to what was said, and to supplement that listening with searching questions. They factored in the effects of weather and season on a patient's intrinsic makeup. They learned to read subtle physical manifestations of disease: the color and texture of a person's tongue, the color, smell, and sediments in the urine, the quality of its bubbles when stirred with a stick. They found remarkably sophisticated methods of reading pulses to assess the health of internal organs.

Many Westerners have difficulty believing that pulse reading and the close examination of urine can offer valuable information to a physician. But it makes intuitive sense that, over centuries of trial and error, cultures find tools that are effective in diagnosing and treating disease. As with natural selection, methods that don't work are abandoned. Those tools that are effective continue to be refined and passed on to future generations, like precious jewels.

Tibetan medicine is particularly well suited to treat illnesses which are chronic or multi-faceted, or diseases that Western practitioners label 'psychosomatic.'

In the West, people often think of Tibetan medicine primarily as a spiritual healing system, but it is important to remember that it is actually a medical science developed through thousands of years of objective analysis, intuition and insight.

TIBETAN MEDICINE AND BUDDHISM

Tibetan medicine and Buddhism are two distinct systems. Buddhist traditions provide the basic cosmology of the Tibetan medical system, a framework for the expression of the interdependence of mind and body and the relationship of a human life to the greater cosmos.

The ability of a Tibetan doctor to bring about healing is linked to that individual's skill, knowledge and depth of experience, but just as important, it is directly connected with that person's wisdom and compassion, wisdom that understands the causes of human suffering, and compassion which seeks to minimize suffering in the world.

QUALITIES OF A SKILLFUL HEALER

A Tibetan physician studies the science and art of healing for five years in a medical college, followed by an additional one year internship with a senior physician. The qualities demanded of a Tibetan doctor include intelligence, compassion, dedication, deep skill, and resourcefulness of body, speech and mind.

To become a skillful healer, a physician must see and feel clearly, without the obstruction or distortion of personal emotions or perceptions. Humility is essential to skillful care, together with a devotion to each individual patient.

In Tibetan medical texts, it is said that the physician should seek to:

• generate compassion on seeing the patients' suffering;

- generate love with a view to helping the patients;
- make no distinction among patients in terms of caste, race or social and economic status;
- become delighted on seeing the patients' recovery;
- generate in one's mind the four immeasurable benevolences (equanimity, love, joy and compassion) when treating a patient.

A Tibetan physician seeks to see the patient as a whole, to gather as precise a picture as possible of the subtle points of balance and imbalance within a person.

THE FIVE ELEMENTS

In the Tibetan medical system, our bodies, like the natural world and all beings living in the world, are considered to be composed of five elements:

earth   (*sa*)
water   (*chu*)
fire   (*mae*)
air   (*loog*)
space   (*namkha*)

Diseases arise from an imbalance of the bodily elements. Medications and remedies which correct imbalances are also made up of the five elements.

When these elements are in balance, the body is in a state of health. If there is a disruption, if there is an unnatural increase or decrease of one element in relation to the other elements, sickness results.

When an imbalance occurs, the body instinctively tries to bring itself back into balance. A simple example: imagine that you're trekking in the Himalayas and your rucksack slides down an icy incline and disappears into a crevasse. The outside temperature plummets; you haven't enough clothing to keep you warm, and the fire of the body diminishes. Your body demands heat and creates it through shivering.

The essence of healing is the body's robust instinct for re-establishing balance. The body and mind know, desire, and find, if possible, what's needed.

The environment is composed of the same five elements as the body; it can either contribute to or challenge human health. As with our bodies, if one element goes seriously out of balance, the result is a natural calamity: a flood, volcanic eruption, hurricane, tornado, or earthquake.

3

THE CAUSES OF SUFFERING & DISEASE

From where does suffering originate? According to Buddhist philosophy, the mind is the root of all suffering. This suffering stems from remote causes that lead to immediate or recent causes.

Remote Causes:

Remote causes are of two types: general and specific.

General:

The general cause of all suffering is rooted in self-grasping ignorance (*bDak-hZin-Marig-pa*). Unless you are a rare, enlightened being, you have the seeds of ignorance within you. You may enjoy prosperity, comfort, and good health, but you're never far removed from the ignorance of self-grasping, just as a bird flying into space, over the mountain, or the sea, or the forest, is never far from her shadow.

Specific:

The specific causes of suffering, or the three mental poisons (*duk sum*), emanate from the ego's self-grasping ignorance. These mental poisons are:

Desire/attachment: (toward an attractive object). The mind takes in sensory information and feels itself at the center of the universe. In our attachment to self (and to our ego-driven opinions, plans, etc.), we ignore the fact that impermanence is omnipresent; we overlook the laws of constant change and transformation; we cling to the objects of our desire. This causes us to suffer. We fall in love, for instance, and become blinded by our attachment, forgetting that life ebbs and flows, expands and contracts, that every meeting contains within it the seeds of separation.

Hatred/anger: (toward a person who is performing something against our wishes and desires). The self-important 'I,' when thwarted or challenged, reacts with anger, aggression, and competitiveness. Angry reactions are based on the illusion that *my* will, *my* desire are all that matter. The effect of this illusion is destructive, both personally and globally.

Close-mindedness/dullness: The mind lacks wisdom, self-awareness and the ability to discriminate between right and wrong, or between virtuous and non-virtuous actions. In its heavy, dull state, the mind is unable to learn from the past, sort out the present, or plan creatively for the future, all of which lead to hasty or ill-considered actions.

Immediate or Recent Causes:

From the three mental poisons, above, come the immediate or recent causes of suffering, called *Nyespas*. The three *Nyespas* are called *Loong*, *Tripa*, and *Badkan*.

The *Nyespas* are powerful forces, vital to the physical body and to our psychological and spiritual selves. While their normal function is to support our well-being, problems occur when they overdevelop in one direction or another. When *Loong, Tripa, and Badkan* are balanced and in the right proportion in their respective sites, we are in good health. But if they are out of balance, or unnaturally increased or disrupted, disease ensues.

From *desire/attachment, Loong* develops. *Loong* generates movement in the bodily functions, mind and speech. When it accompanies the *Tripa* or hot element, it helps warm the body. When it accompanies the *Badkan* or cold element, it helps chill the body. Because it generates movement, it is a necessary condition for the onset of any illness. As it diffuses through all parts of the body, it can disrupt both the hot and cold elements. Therefore, *Loong* is the basic catalyst of all disease.

From *hatred/anger, Tripa* (burning, inflammation) develops. All 'hot diseases' (septic conditions, inflammations, and the elevation of body temperature) originate from *Tripa:* imbalanced *Tripa* burns the bodily constituents. It is in the nature of fire to burn upwards. So with *Tripa*. Its site is in the lower part of body, but complications arising from it are often found in the upper part of the body. There is not a single 'hot disease' not originating from Tripa.

From *close-mindedness/dullness, Badkan* (cold element) develops. Some examples of 'cold diseases' are anemia, chills, chronically cold extremities, frequent urination, all of which originate when the body contains too much *Badkan*. Disrupted *Badkan* lowers the digestive heat. It carries earth and water elements and creates problems in the lower part of the body, even though it resides in the upper part of the body. This is akin to snow melting and flooding a valley below. There is not a single 'cold disease' not originating from Badkan.

Loong overdevelops because of insatiable desire, *Tripa* when anger becomes a ruling force, *Badkan* when close-mindedness or ignorance predominate. Like all strong forces, they have the power to both support and do harm. (A fire warms us and helps us cook our food; but out of control, it can cut through healthy forests and sweep homes into oblivion.)

For illness to occur, the propelling condition must be there. If you have a seed of rice in your pocket, the seed sprouts if the conditions are right. Our body carries the seeds of disease within it, but it is impossible for fruit to grow from the seed without the condition.

A boil on your forehead is an example of an effect arising from the seed of disease. A Tibetan medical practitioner will seek to understand what has caused the eruption. This points to one of the fundamental precepts of Tibetan medicine: one must treat the fundamental cause. If one treats only the effect, a symptom will manifest again, perhaps in a different form, perhaps more seriously the next time. It may lie dormant for a time, but an effect of some sort will reappear.

THE THREE NYESPAS

Loong, the Mobile Force

The essence of life is movement: the everlasting cycles of birth to death. Ocean tides rise and fall; the seasons move inexorably forward—spring, summer, fall, winter, and back to spring. Every living thing moves. Sap rises, new leaves spring from tightly closed buds, flowers bloom, birds migrate, rivers rush with new rains.

Time never pauses. No sooner do we think of this moment as 'present' than it is past. In the same way, our thoughts are in constant motion. One thought becomes a doorway to another and another. Even mountains, a symbol of solidity, evolve over time. The great Himalayas move upward at a rate of about 5 mm per year. And they fall away. Rocks cascade into river valleys, soil washes away, the faces of mountains change.

All movement in humans—body, mind and speech—comes from *Loong.* Its force is responsible for the movements of our hands and legs, for the movement of every organ in the body and its nervous system. Every second of every day, we breathe in and out, our chests rise and fall, our blood moves. We process constantly changing information through our senses, emotions move through us, our sexual passions are aroused, we digest food and eliminate waste. In its normal, balanced state, *Loong* maintains the body.

Loong is connected to the mental poison of desire, lust and attachment, and it is thought to reside in the lower part of the body around the genital organs, hips and waist. One translation for *Loong* is wind, an unseen but powerful force. Given that it is responsible for all movement in the body, diseases begin and end with *Loong* and are intensified by the presence of this force.

When *Loong* is in an unbalanced state, a person may become irritable, mentally and physically restless, talk excessively, suffer tension and stiffness around the neck, or become anxious or depressed. Nights may be disturbed or sleepless.

Other symptoms include: frequent yawning and sighs (the body attempting to release excess accumulaton of *Loong*), dizziness, hazy vision, ringing in the ears, pain and stiffness in the body, tightness. There may be dry heaves, or chills and shivering. When too much *Loong* force is present, the mind feels light, unstable, changeable; it becomes difficult to stick to one's decisions or keep one's word. At times, the mind becomes unhinged: a person is disconnected from reality and experiences hallucinations or delirium—laughing, singing, dancing, crying.

Tibetan medical practitioners consider disorders of the nervous system to be an imbalance in *Loong* , whereas other medical systems consider many of these disorders to be psychological.

Physical exhaustion, or mental stresses and pressures leading to worry and depression, provoke an imbalance in *Loong*. Other causes of *Loong* imbalance include the following: eating poorly or fasting excessively, ingesting too many foods or beverages having a bitter taste, exposure to cold wind, immoderate sexual intercourse, lifting loads that are too heavy, or withholding or applying pressure for natural urges (defecation, urination, sneezing).

Consciousness and *Loong* are interdependent. It is said that consciousness without *Loong* is like a man who cannot move his legs, while *Loong* without consciousness is like a horse with no eyes. Taming the mind and keeping it happy and content helps to insure that *Loong* maintains a proper balance and does its part to promote good physical health.

Tripa, the Sun at the Center of our Solar System

Without the sun, life as we know it, would perish. Each winter, people who live in northern climates experience the effect of cold on the body & mind. Spring comes again, and the heat of the sun warms the skin and bones. Life bursts forth; our minds become filled with joy and gratefulness. This is the power of the sun.

Tripa is the force in our bodies that delivers heat. It resides in the middle part of the body, in the area of the liver, gall bladder and small intestine. Its pathways are the secretory and endocrine systems, and it is linked with the blood, perspiration, eyes, and intestines. *Tripa* is responsible for a good complexion, for helping the skin glow. It also facilitates good eyesight. Most importantly, it is necessary for healthy digestion and is therefore at the root of all good health. The Tibetan medical text says: "The stomach is like a field; one must maintain its heat, just as a farmer who desires an abundant harvest, keeps the field fertile." If the digestive fire is in good working order, the body can digest, absorb and make good use of nutrients for preserving health.

Eating at a time of day when the body wants to shut down and be quiet, or eating in excess, makes one prone to digestive disturbances. In Tibet, there is a saying, "While you are a guest at a party, do not forget that the stomach is yours, even though the food is served by others." Overeating and drinking can lead to disorders of the body and mind.

In its balanced, positive form, *Tripa* gives us courage and fortitude and encourages us to think ahead and to approach endeavors with intelligence and foresight. If *Tripa* is out of balance, however, it launches us into aggression and competitiveness. The ego becomes all-consuming, a blind, petty tyrant lording it over others and causing grief and suffering. *Tripa* in its unbalanced state is linked to the 'mental poison' of hatred or anger. Anger in turn is fueled by the illusion that the ego is all important: my desire, *my* needs, *my* will, *my* opinions, *my* plans—if you're not with me, you're against me.

When people are in the grip of unbalanced *Tripa*, the body temperature rises. Like flames that begin at the foundation of a house and rise to the roof, anger causes the face to perspire and grow red with the heat of thwarted ego. *Tripa* in its most unbalanced state is destructive at a personal and global level.

Some causes of *Tripa* disease are the following: overuse of very rich foods (meat and butter) or alcohol; allowing the mind to rage; sleeping during midday or under the scorching heat of the sun; experiencing a serious accident; or doing very strenuous physical work or exercise, especially when the body is unaccustomed to it.

Symptoms of *Tripa* imbalance may include headaches, elevation of body temperature, a bitter or sour taste in the mouth, dryness in the nostrils, excessive thirst, diarrhea, a piercing, localized pain, excessive perspiration.

To keep *Tripa* in a balanced state and to assist the regulation of the digestive fire, the following advice is helpful:

- Do not eat unless you feel hungry.

- Do not drink unless you are thirsty.

- Do not eat when you feel thirsty.

- Do not drink when you feel hungry.

Badkan, the Cool, Lunar Power

The meaning of *Badkan* is 'phlegmatic' and 'cold.' It combines the elements of earth and water and produces a moistening, cooling quality, counteracting the heat of *Tripa* and keeping our body temperature in balance. It moistens the organs, lubricates joints, develops firmness in the body. It supports that part of our mind which is patient, tolerant and relaxed.

Badkan is connected to the moon, to the tides, and to the gravitational pull on our bodies. Its power is transmitted through liquid mediums. Most body tissues—including muscle, skin and body organs—contain over 70% water.

The seat of *Badkan* lies in the upper part of the body, predominantly in the brain. An overabundance of this cool element causes dullness, ignorance, and lack of understanding. When the mind becomes dull and closed, self-awareness disappears. One cannot grasp ideas, assimilate or process information, or make good decisions or morally defensible judgments. Clarity and insight are blocked.

When *Badkan's* cold property is elevated, the digestive heat begins to slacken. An impaired digestive system prevents us from assimilating food and leads to an accumulation of undigested particles of food, which can become toxic in the body. With too much *Badkan*, normal circulation of the blood will be negatively affected, leading to skin eruptions, respiratory or cardiovascular problems. A runny nose, cough, indigestion, asthma, and swelling of the legs can often be traced to *Badkan*.

With a *Badkan* disease, the gums and tongue become pale, and one's taste sensations become dull. The body feels heavy, lethargic and drowsy, and the extremities are cold to the touch. A person may experience pain in the kidney and waist region. These conditions become worse during rainy periods, evening and morning, and immediately after eating.

Although *Badkan* resides in the upper part of the body, complications often occur in the lower part of the body (stomach and kidney). An excess of *Badkan* in the body produces a sensation of general heaviness and lethargy, excessive phlegm and mucus, a feeling of cold, and unnaturally heavy sleep.

Some causes of *Badkan* imbalance are the following: overuse of bitter, sweet, heavy, or cold foods; eating unripened fruits, or vegetables that have grown stale or wilted; eating too much raw or undercooked food; drinking cold goat's milk, or eating goat's meat or yogurt; too much oil, fat or butter; drinking cold water or tea that has not been well-boiled.

A *Badkan* imbalance can arise from overeating (or eating before the previous food has been digested); lying down immediately after eating; sleeping in the daytime; lying on wet ground; swimming in the cold season; and not dressing warmly enough.

Physical exercise is helpful in treating *Badkan* disorders. One excellent form of exercise consists of 'prostrations' (*Chhag*), a Tibetan form of exercise and devotion. To do a prostration, begin in a standing position, palms together in front of the chest. Crouch down to a squatting position, then kneel forward. Keeping the body as close to the ground as possible, with the palms sliding forward in front, stretch out to your full length. Then pull the body back to the kneeling position and return to starting position. Ten to fifteen prostrations every morning and evening are very good for balancing the *Badkan*.

LOONG, TRIPA & BADKAN PERSONALITY
TRAITS

People are born with particular natures, inherited from their parents' dispositions, propensities, or from the conditions of a mother's pregnancy. Given the complexity of a human being, people rarely represent a pure *Loong, Tripa,* or *Badkan* type. However, one can distinguish between seven gross categories of people:

Loong type
Tripa type
Badkan type
Loong/Tripa type
Badkan/Tripa type
Badkan/Loong type
Loong/Tripa/Badkan type

These categories help a physician establish guideposts and conduct accurate diagnoses and treatments.

Loong nature: *Loong* personalities are talkative and love music, singing and laughter. Their favorite tastes are sweet, hot and sour. They typically have a thin and slightly stooped body and a bluish complexion. Their joints may crack when moving, and their bodies do not tolerate cold well. They generally sleep lightly, for shorter hours than other types, and often are easily distracted. They tend to have a restless nature, moving here and there.

Tripa nature: *Tripa* types generally have a high metabolism and are often hungry and thirsty. They often have a reddish complexion and perspire easily. They are intelligent, competitive and proud. Their favorite tastes are sweet, bitter and astringent. During pregnancy, a mother increases the chances of having a *Tripa* child if she eats rich, or hot, spicy foods, drinks alcohol, engages in heavy physical exertion, acts out aggression, or carries the child predominantly in the autumn.

Badkan nature: *Badkan* people are often tall, with an upright carriage. They have a whitish complexion and can tolerate hunger, thirst and heat. They are slow to become angry and generally deal with stress more easily than other types. They enjoy helping others and tend to live a long life. They tend to sleep heavily, and to be slow in speech and movement. They have a preference for sweet, hot, and sour tastes and may be overweight. If a mother during pregnancy eats a lot of raw, cold food, or carries her child during the cold, wet season, the fetus will be influenced toward *Badkan* nature.

THE EFFECT OF EXTERNAL ELEMENTS ON
LOONG, TRIPA, & BADKAN

In their natural cycles, diseases accumulate, arise and pacify.

Loong diseases tend to arise during the rainy season and worsen at twilight and dawn.

Tripa diseases often arise during autumn and are intensified at midday and midnight.

Spring heightens the tendency toward *Badkan* disease, which worsens in the evening and morning.

Babies and children, whose bodies and minds are not yet fully developed, are more susceptible to *Badkan* disorders. Adults (the stage in life when people are likely to experience the greatest pride-induced anger and aggression) are prone to *Tripa* disorders. Elderly people, whose sensory organs, appetite and digestion tend to diminish, are susceptible to *Loong* diseases.

EXTERNAL CONDITIONS WHICH CREATE DISEASE

Together with the imbalance of *Nyespas*, the Tibetan medical system holds that the two major causes of disease are diet and lifestyle. In addition, environmental conditions plus what Tibetan practitioners refer to as 'evil spirits,' can affect our resilience in the face of disease.

Diet:

Diet is a major factor in creating good health. To promote optimum health, we must balance the five elements as they exist in food and ensure that we do not misuse or overuse particular foods. There are six distinct tastes that are thought to be manifestations of the five elements.

Formation of any material needs all the five elements: the earth element forms the base, water assembles, fire ripens, air assists in the further development, and the space element helps the rest grow expansively. All the five elemental materials have tastes; these tastes differ because of the predominance of one or more elements in their makeup, as follows:

Taste	Predominant Elements
Sweet	Earth and Water
Sour	Earth and Fire
Salty	Fire and Water
Bitter	Water and Air
Hot	Air and Fire
Astringent	Earth and Air

Sweet, sour and salty are considered superior tastes; the latter three are considered inferior tastes. All supplement our bodies' needs and cause suffering if *misuse, disuse,* or *overuse* of particular foods occur:

Overuse occurs through an excess taste of any type of food or beverage or an overuse of sweet or salty, etc.; heavy, indigestible foods at night; too much raw salad eaten in the evening, at the onset of the cold, *Badkan* period of the day.

Disuse through excessive fasting, starvation, eating or drinking too little.

Misuse through eating when the body wants to shut down; eating contaminated food; combining foods that have contradictory effects (milk with citrus, or cold water with fatty foods—cold slows down the digestive processes needed for digesting heavy foods).

Lifestyle & Behaviors:

As with food, a healthy lifestyle leads to good health. If you wish to live a disease free life, it is important to be aware of *choelam,* or the activities of body, mind and speech. Misuse, disuse or overuse of body, mind and speech create the conditions for sickness.

• Body:

Overuse through pushing the body and bodily parts to do more than they can tolerate (such as physical exertion, or overusing or straining the sensory organs).

Disuse through lack of sensory activities or physical movement.

Misuse through neglecting the body, not valuing and caring for it; smoking, engaging in addictive behaviors; lifting things that are too heavy, pushing the body beyond endurance; subjecting the body to long-term stress; not getting adequate sleep; engaging in non-virtuous physical acts (e.g. stealing, killing, adultery or other actions leading to guilt and mental discomfort), or withholding or pressuring natural urges, such as defecation and urination).

- Mind:

Overuse through thinking too much; mental stress, tension, anxiety, or thinking without understanding or insight or realization; holding an opinion too tightly (over-attachment to an idea); obsessing over things you desire (over-attachment to things).

Disuse through an absent mind; lack of concentration, thoughts and concern.

Misuse through negative thoughts that destroy calm or peace or friendships; wrong motivation; non-virtuous thoughts, temptations, harmful thoughts.

- Speech:

Overuse through talking too much, too long, or too loud.

Disuse through dullness.

Misuse through lying; gossiping; creating unrest between friends; talking about people behind their backs.

In making lifestyle choices, *think* before you speak, before you decide, and before you act. Ask, how will it affect me and others? A thoughtful approach to speaking, decision-making and action leads to peace and harmony and helps create good health, not only at an individual but also at the global level.

Environmental / Seasonal Conditions:

Three potential defects are connected with climate conditions:
- excessive amounts (of cold, heat, rain, etc.)
- amounts below normal expectations
- conditions unsuitable to the season

Our lives are dependent on environmental conditions; they need cold from winter, heat from summer, and rain— not too much nor too little or unsuited to the season. If an apple tree is coaxed into bud by an unseasonably warm spell and then gets nipped by cold, the tree will weaken and produce less fruit. Like the tree, we develop internal expectations for cold, rain, sun, and warmth; if there's too much, too little, or unexpected manifestations, our health and resilience are affected.

Evil Spirits:

This term can easily be misunderstood by Westerners. 'Evil spirits' are best thought of as describing inner psychological processes: negative thoughts, bitterness and resentment, something troubling or unresolved. Evil spirits develop in our minds; they prevent rejuvenation and block our ability to experience the world with hope and joy. In an enlightened mind, there is no 'I' or ego, and therefore no evil spirits. Most minds, however, are unenlightened and therefore subject to the storms of the ego. Evil spirits are a shorthand way of speaking about the despair, anger, or fear that accompanies ego blindness and ignorance.

The adverse affect that evil spirits have on our health is another way of speaking about the body-mind connection: the ways that emotional stress, wear and tear, or avoidance can impact our physical well-being.

A Tibetan lama may perform rites and rituals to rid a person of evil spirits. For the body to respond and react positively, the patient must have deep faith and believe in the remedy offered for purification.

4

DIAGNOSIS OF DISEASE

There are three major diagnostic methods that a Tibetan physician calls upon: visual examination, examination by touch, and examination by questioning and listening.

• Visual (*tahwa*):

When a patient comes through the door, the physician closely observes the person's body structure, complexion, speech and behavior: e.g., is the person hyper, low energy, aggressive, anxious, depressed? It is also important to examine visually the external sensory organs which give clear information concerning their relative internal organs, to be aware of this information transmitted by what are called 'flower-like symptoms.' For example, liver problems can be understood by observing, among other things, a patient's jaundiced eyes. Kidney problems can be detected through tinnitus, deafness, or humming in the ears. Lung disease through nasal blockage and runny nose. Stammering and cracked tongues may reveal heart problems. The spleen manifests its disorders through cracked and coated lips, among other things.

The color of a patient's tongue also yields useful information. If a person is suffering from a *Loong* disease, the tongue will be dry and reddish, with small red pimples. In a *Tripa* disease, the tongue will have a thick, yellowish coating, and the saliva will have a bitter taste. In a *Badkan* disease, the tongue will appear pale and thick, with the impression of teeth at the edges. There will also be evidence of excessive mucus and phlegm.

A urine sample reveals the following:

Loong disease: the urine will be thin and watery. When stirred, there will be big bubbles ('the size of a yak's eye'), and there may appear fine sediments, like the hair of a goat. There is no taste.

Tripa disease: presents urine of a reddish yellow color, bad smelling, with a lot of steam. When stirred, small bubbles disappear immediately. Sediments appear like fine white wool. The taste is bitter.

Badkan disease: the urine will appear whitish in color without much steam or smell. The taste is sweet or sour. Stirring reveals tiny tips of white—like horse hair. Foam or sticky saliva-like bubbles will also be produced.

• Examination by touch (*rekpa*):

Pulse reading is a highly refined art which takes years to fully master. It is one of the most essential diagnostic tools of Tibetan medicine. The physician 'reads' the pulse on the radial artery of the wrist. The index finger is placed near the joint and lightly touches the skin; the middle finger adds a little more pressure, and the ring finger applies even more pressure. The state of each major organ in the body can be read through the pulse:

The left hand radial artery of a male patient felt by the right hand of a physician indicates the following:

Reading Finger:	Corresponding Organs:
Index	Heart / Small Intestine
Middle	Spleen / Stomach
Ring	Left Kidney / Reproductive Organ

The right hand radial pulse of a male patient felt by the left hand of physician indicates:

Reading Finger:	Corresponding Organs:
Index	Lung / Large Intestine
Middle	Liver / Gall Bladder
Ring	Right Kidney / Urinary Bladder

In the case of a female patient, the organs corresponding to the physician's index fingers are opposite of those for male patients. The left hand pulse indicates the lung and large intestine; the right hand pulse indicates the heart and small intestine.

A *Loong* pulse is floating and superficial. When pressure is applied, it disappears like a balloon on water. Sometimes you will feel dropped beats.

The *Tripa* pulse is thin, tight and fast.

The *Badkan* pulse is sinking, slow and weak.

Studying the characteristics of the pulse alone is not enough. It is essential to think of the patient as a unique web of interconnected forces.

• Examination by questioning (*driwa*):

In Tibetan culture, Mount Kailash, a 22,000 peak located in a remote area in the far Western part of Tibet, is considered the cosmic center of the universe. Tibetans do not scale the mountain or carry trophies away from it; they show their devotion by doing *kora* around the base of the mountain, through walking and prayer.

Similarly, a Tibetan physician is expected to practice medicine, not for ego gratification or glory but to be of service to one's fellow human beings. Tibetan doctors are taught to enter into the physician-patient relationship with devotion, openness and care, and to treat patients with humility and compassion.

In this spirit, a Tibetan doctor develops the capacity to ask searching, intelligent questions and to listen under the surface of a person's answers to achieve a more complete understanding of the causes, symptoms and location of diseases. A physician asks for the signs and symptoms of the disease, the site of pain, the duration of the illness, the cause of sickness from a patient's point of view.

By knowing the cause of disease, the physician can specify the particular *Nyespas*. The site of the pain indicates the location of disease, and the signs and symptoms confirm the specific disorder.

It is rare to find any illness that emanates from simply *Loong, Tripa or Badkan*. More commonly, the *Nyespas* work in concert with each other; if one *Nyespa* has lost its footing, all three are affected and out of balance. Adding to the complexity, each person carries with them a unique and complex set of characteristics.

Symptoms by themselves cannot be relied upon to reveal the whole picture. A headache, for instance, can be caused by *Tripa* rising upward into the head like a flame; it is also possible that imbalanced *Loong* has caused the headache by pushing *Tripa* upwards. Depending upon the cause, the treatment must be different. In addition, the location of pain can be deceptive. The pain is a symptom, and the root of the illness may lie elsewhere.

Because Tibetan medicine delves beneath the surface of symptoms, it is particularly effective for treating chronic diseases (*gChong-nad*). Diseases such as arthritis, asthma, diabetes, rheumatism, liver diseases and illnesses related to the nervous and digestive systems can be effectively treated through a combination of medicine, and prescribed diet and lifestyle changes. Since a sluggish digestion can cause the build-up of toxins which create growths and tumors, edema, or spleen or liver enlargement, the digestive system is of particular importance when treating chronic diseases.

TREATMENT ALTERNATIVES

If the mind is the root of all suffering, taming the mind's excesses and distortions and ego desires are at the root of all treatment. Buddhist practices (and other spiritual traditions) provide a path that leads in this direction.

Treatments in Tibetan medicine are based on changes to diet or lifestyle, augmented with medicines and other therapies.

• **Diet:**

Advice given to a person suffering from *Loong* diseases includes the addition of nutritious, warm food, plus foods which have a sweet, sour, or salty taste. For a *Tripa* disease, light, cool food is helpful, like yogurt, light cereal, or fruit juices with sweet, bitter or astringent tastes. For a *Badkan* disease, relief comes from food that is hot and light in nature, with a sour, astringent and pungent taste.

One of the healthiest things one can do early every morning before eating is to drink a cup of boiled water. It is also good to do this in the evening, just after sunset. There are a number of benefits that accrue from this simple action. The cold *Badkan* force predominates in the mornings and evenings. Boiled water helps to warm the body and balance the cold. For people who frequently suffer from colds and coughs, it is a useful preventive measure. Boiled water helps cleanse the body of accumulated mucus in the throat and lungs. And it is very good for digestion, supporting the digestive fire.

- **Lifestyle:**

For a person affected by *Loong* disease, a physician is likely to recommend that the person spend time with close, companionable, kind friends. The environment should be meditative, quiet, and free from disturbance and stress.

A person with *Tripa* disease will find relief in a cooling place, near a river or by the seashore, or under shady trees, free from situations which provoke anger.

Badkan disturbances are relieved by prostration (*Chhag*), physical exercise, sunshine, and warmth.

- **Medicines:**

A Tibetan physician will typically give a patient several different types of medication for use each day. This differs from single focus drugs common in Western medicine. In Tibetan medicine, one type of medicine may address the primary challenge while the other medicines ensure that the body stays in balance. Tibetan medicines are traditionally comprised of anywhere from ten to over a hundred ingredients.

Some Tibetan medicines require at least a day to take effect, while others take less time. Typically, Tibetan medicines are slower acting than medicines taken by Western patients. Behind the slower, steadier application of Tibetan medicine is the knowledge that medicines must be assimilated by the entire digestive process.

The strength of a medicine is also of the utmost importance. Problems can arise when a strong medicine is used for minor diseases, or a weak medicine for serious illnesses. It is said that if a load meant for a yak is placed on a sheep, it may break the sheep's legs or back; if a load meant for a sheep is placed on a yak, the yak won't feel anything.

- **External Therapies:**

These include medicinal baths, oil massage, fomentations, both hot and cold, and in special cases, bloodletting (for diseases originating from a disorder of *Tripa* and blood), and moxibustion (for diseases originating from *Loong* and *Badkan*).

The simplest prescriptions for creating everyday health and vitality are as follows:

Think before you speak.
Think before you eat.
Think before you decide.
Think before you act.

Smile at least three times a day.

5

IN SUMMARY

Buddhist teachings offer freedom from endless desire, anger, and confusion. A skillful physician is a messenger between a suffering world and a world that is balanced and healthy and free from common human afflictions. Tibetan physicians are highly attuned to the close relationship between the mind and body, and to the ways that negative perceptions and emotions manifest in imbalance and ill-health. Much of their efforts are therefore directed toward protecting the body from disease by helping patients to create the habits of mind which free them from distortion and unhappiness.

Our small egos see our beings as the center of the universe, competitive, separate from everyone and everything. In truth, our bodies and minds are profoundly linked to the rest of creation. This is the starting point of Tibetan medicine. We do not exist as independent beings, but as interdependent beings in a subtle, vast, ocean of being.

As one of the oldest known medical traditions in the world, the Tibetan medical system is steadily expanding and developing across the world. In 1960, shortly after China's invasion of Tibet, His Holiness the Dalai Lama established Men-Tsee-Khang, the Tibetan Medical and Astrological Institute in Dharamsala, India. The Institute now has 42 branches and over 100 doctors working in India. As Westerners increasingly experience the benefit of Tibetan medicine, there is a growing interest in Tibetan consultations and clinics in the West. A number of Tibetan doctors, Dr. Pema Dorjee included, have traveled extensively in Europe, and North and South America.

In addition to clinical training and practice, the Tibetan Medical and Astrological Institute has a clinical research department, where research into treatments for diabetes, asthma, cancer, and other chronic illnesses is ongoing.

The weaving together of eastern and western medical perspectives offers the possibility for healing that neither tradition can accomplish on its own. Dr. Bernard Lown, a cardiologist on the faculty of the Harvard Medical School who won the Nobel Prize for his work with Physicians for Social Responsibility, said, "I was trained as a classical cardiologist, and I was initially in my career one of the big promoters of medical technology and technologic solutions, but on much reflection as I get older, I sense ... the loss of community and the loss of social connectedness which gives meaning to life." Western medicine has offered much to the world. And Tibetan medicine, with its holistic approach and unique physician-patient partnership has proven effective in healing certain types of illnesses that still mystify Western practitioners.

Although clinics specializing in Tibetan medicine are

difficult to find outside of Tibet, India, Nepal and Bhutan because of the challenges of language differences, cultural differences and government regulation, the influence of Tibetan medicine has expanded and continues to do so.

China's invasion and occupation of Tibet has had tragic repercussions for Tibet's people and culture. One of the few silver linings in this cloud of sorrow has been the increasing availability of Tibet's cultural wisdom, which was largely out of sight until the 1950's. One can hope that physicians and health professionals in Tibet and the West will take every opportunity to further the numbers of mutual exchanges: through lectures, international conferences, training sessions, internships and residencies—interactions which will create benefits to patients through the broadening of outlook, perspective, diagnostic tools and treatment options.

40

About the Authors:

Dr. Pema Dorjee was nine years old when his family fled Tibet. In 1960, he enrolled in the Tibetan Refugee School in Darjeeling, India, and graduated in 1968. He attended the Tibetan Medical College in Dharamsala, beginning in 1969, and completed his studies in 1974, studying under the renowned scholar, Dr. Barshi Phuntsog Wangyal and interning with the highly skilled Dr. Yeshi Dhonden. He was posted to Dharamsala, Mcleod Ganj, then Delhi, Arunachal Pradesh, Calcutta, Silguri, and back to Dharamsala. He served as General Secretary of the Institute and as first Chairman of the Medical Council and is presently the Director of the Research Department.

Dr. Dorjee has lectured at universities and held workshops and consultations in a number of countries, including England, Kazakhstan, U.S. Chile, Columbia and Brazil, and written articles published in the U.S. and U.K. *The Spiritual Medicine of Tibet: Heal Your Spirit, Heal Yourself*, co-authored with Janet Jones and Terence Moore, was published in London in 2005.

Pema Dorjee sees many hundreds of patients a year in Dharamsala, Ladakh, Calcutta, Darjeeling, and in Western countries. About his work, he says, "Through this path, I have seen many walks of life—famous people, political leaders, and very poor people. Love and compassion is at the heart of my work. To be able to relieve suffering gives me the highest satisfaction. I have never felt anything lacking in what I do."

Dr. Dorjee, one of the most senior and renowned Tibetan medical practioners outside Tibet, is married to Dr.

Yeshi Khando Dorjee, who practices Tibetan medicine in Majnu-ka-Tila in Delhi. Their eldest daughter, Tenzin Yangkyi, graduated with a B.Sc. from St. Joseph College, Darjeeling and holds a degree in Tibetan Medicine and Surgery from the Institute of Higher Tibetan Studies in Saranat, Varanasi. Their younger daughter, Tenzin Choeying, holds a BA in Political Science (Honours) from Delhi University and has recently graduated from the Tibetan Medical College in Dharamsala.

Eleanor Lincoln Morse lives on Peaks Island in the northeastern United States. She has written two novels, *Chopin's Garden* and *An Unexpected Forest,* which won the 2008 Independent Publisher Book Award for best northeast regional fiction. She teaches writing through Spalding University's brief-residency Master of Fine Arts in Writing Program in Louisville, Kentucky, and lives with John Moncure Wetterau, a writer of fiction, non-fiction and poetry.

John and Eleanor have three children and two grandchildren between them. They have also become sponsors to a seventeen-year old Tibetan girl, who graduated from Gopalpur School in Himachal Pradesh, northern India in 2009.